HOW TO CONTROL YOUR SEXUAL URGE

TABLE OF CONTENT.

INTRODUCTION

Sexual response is a deeply rooted key physiological condition found throughout the species. The study of sexuality in animals is a complex topic that could be approached from different perspectives, given that it relies on the interplay between nervous, endocrine, and genetic factors. In humans, sexual behavior is influenced by cultural settings requiring dynamic behavioral adaptation. Therefore, a multisystem interaction is necessary to guarantee both features and the more complex functions typical of humans. Neural structures engaged in sexual behavior are located throughout the nervous system, both in its central and in its peripheral divisions. Detection of multimodal sexual stimuli involves sensory processing that merges with experiences to trigger autonomic as well as proper motor responses under an overwhelming cognitive control. To date, although the neural mechanisms underlying desire, arousal, and orgasm are the same in both males and females, sexual responses, however, are different between genders.

WHAT ARE URGES?

Urges are intense physical responses.They are the biological, psychological,and social aspect of addition coming together. Urges are a normal part of life and not unhealthy. It's what you do about the urge that matters.

HOW TO OVERCOME SEXUAL URGE.

Sex is a beautiful way to express your love and affection to someone you love. However, sexual desires can be a problem sometimes. For example, having an affair can cause a lot of pain to all parties involved, especially the one that got cheated on. Partners who cheated would usually say that they "didn't mean it" or that "the sex didn't mean anything."

Sex is a normal part of human nature, but uncontrolled sexual desires can put you in situations you never wanted to be in. Sexual desires need to be controlled. If not, they will cause dysfunction in your relationships and mental health.

This article will give you tips on how you can manage your compulsive sexual behavior. Read along and learn ways to control these sexual impulses and where you can ask for help when you can't control them. Sexual urges can be a problem when they start affecting your relationships and sexual behavior.

Understanding your sex drive.

Libido is a simplified term for the desire to engage in sexual activity. Humans, just like animals, need to have sex to reproduce. Libido is rooted deeply in our biology to encourage us to produce another human being.

There is no such thing as "normal levels" for sex drive. Some couples feel like having sex every day. Some would have it once a week. How often you have sex with your partner depends on your agreement with each other. If your partner agrees to have sex anytime and both of you get satisfied, your libido levels are normal.

Having a high libido can become a problem when sexual desires feel out of control and become compulsions. Some factors, including social and psychological ones, can control our libido levels.

Here are some factors that affect our libido levels:

Level of fatigue

Having a history of sexual abuse

Depression and anxiety

Estrogen and testosterone levels

Abuse of drugs and alcohol

Religious norms

Quality of relationship

Compulsive Sexual Behavior

This behavior is commonly known as sex addiction. It is a hypersexuality disorder with an excessive preoccupation with sexual thoughts and fantasies. The sexual urge becomes the major focus in life that negatively impacts a person's mental health.

Sex addiction is a psychiatric disorder that has negative results on the patient's psychological and physical health. Clinical treatments for these kinds of psychological disorders are not yet formalized, and they aren't directly listed under DSM-5. However, medical centers are already catering to patients suffering from such disorders.

A major characteristic of this disorder is the repetitive sexual act despite adverse consequences. These activities are self-destructive to the point where patients already neglect their health, self-care, and intimacy with their spouse.

Do you know someone you consider a sex addict? Here are some signs that they may be struggling with a high sex drive:

They are unable to achieve sexual satisfaction. No matter how often they have sex or masturbate, they seem incapable of lowering their sexual energy. They feel like they are unable to get the amount of sex they desire.

They can't stop sexual activity. Whether they are watching porn or having sex with a stranger, they can't stop doing it even if it has already affected their social relationships.

They do "it" all the time. They start sacrificing their work, sleep, and social relationships for sex. But always feel empty and unsatisfied after having sex.

They are using sex as an escape from life. These people always find reasons to justify their sexual compulsions. They even sneak around and lie to people who care about them.

How to Control Sexual Desire: Ways to Control Your Sexual Urges

A married man with uncontrolled sexual urges tends to give in and book a sex worker to gain feelings of relief and fulfillment. The consequences of these unhealthy desires are infidelity and adultery.

High libido only becomes a problem when you start ditching work or cheating on a partner because of it. In other words, when these unwanted sexual feelings are not restrained, they could destroy relationships and families. Here are some ways to control them:

1, Identify the Things That Trigger Sexual Urges
To avoid tempting situations, you must first identify what triggers your sexual desires. They may be prompted by sexual fantasies and imaginations in which your physical body reacts by being aroused.

Remain alert and take time to do a self-assessment. Know the environment or the time of the day when you usually start thinking about sex. Try to determine if there is a pattern in your behavior and break it by changing your lifestyle. Finding a new hobby can also help you focus on something rather than indulging yourself with your sexual thoughts.

2. Know the First Line of Defense
Some easily give in to their sexual urges and would easily find release through masturbation. This is okay, but not if you are in the middle of a meeting or during working hours.

Be sure to know the first thing to do when erotic thoughts and feelings arise. Interrupt the sexual fantasies by stopping yourself right there. Avoid eye contact with someone in the office who arouses you sexually. Stop those sexual thoughts from growing in your mind immediately.

Have a list of what you will gain from not giving in to temptations and stick to them. Know how to channel your sexual energy into something creative and spiritual.

3. Avoid Watching Porn
Nowadays, this billion-dollar industry has become more difficult to ignore. Viewing porn has become socially acceptable and accessible through the web. Exposure to porn sites triggers urges to masturbate, so try to use filters on your laptops or cellphones to block these kinds of content.

4. Abstain from Drugs and Alcohol
Sexual activity under the influence of alcohol or drugs is linked to a higher risk of unhealthy sexual behavior. You lose your inhibitions when you're drunk or high, which could also mean losing control over your sexual urges.

The link between sex addiction and substance abuse is a co-occurring disorder. They work hand in hand. Addiction to both sex and drugs or alcohol can worsen into criminal behaviors such as rape and sexual assault.

Stop yourself from going to places or attending parties that you know might become problematic. Control your drinks and know your alcohol tolerance.

5. Talk to Others Who Can Help
Being aware of your body and knowing that you have a high sex drive is nothing to feel bad about. It is normal if one party has a higher libido than the other person in the relationship.

Your sexual relationship with your partner is not over yet. You could always talk to a psychosexual and relationship therapist to help you sort things out.

Is Having a High Sex Drive a Problem?
Having a high libido is not a problem if you don't feel like your urges are controlling you. An increase in sexual desire is usually experienced by young people going through hormonal surges. When older, having a high libido can be a symptom of a medical illness or a side effect of the medication you're taking.

Studies show that higher libido levels are usually found in men than in women. This male versus female myth is a common stereotype when we talk about sex drive. However, research suggests that heterosexual women are often more interested in sex than their male counterparts.

Having a higher sex drive is normal. We should not feel embarrassed about it. There are is no precise way to measure sex drive. Only you can tell if your libido is higher than your partner's sexual desire or if you have a higher sex drive now compared to a few months ago.

Having a higher sex drive could be a good sign that you're getting good sex. That's why your body craves it more. It could also mean having lower stress levels and being capable of giving yourself a break and enjoying pleasurable sexual feelings.

Sexual impulses may fluctuate over the years. It is most of the time linked to distress and relationship issues. Some cases of lower libido are caused by overfamiliarity with your partner and your relationship. It could also be caused by unresolved arguments and frequent conflict with your spouse that you lose the drive for sex.

Here are some ways that can help you boost your libido:

Stop or swap your current medications. Medicines like birth control pills, antidepressants, and beta-blockers have side effects of lowering sex drive. Have your meds reviewed by your doctor and ask for alternatives for these medications.

Eat food that increases libido. There are some natural foods that help increase sex drive. Raw oysters and chocolates are known as edible aphrodisiacs.

Boost your sexual confidence. Established intimate relationships can result in higher sexual confidence. Sex is undeniably an enjoyable activity between two consenting adults. Being a part of an intimate relationship means that both parties are satisfied sexually that they want to stay in it.

Take time to relax. Stress can destroy your sex life. Give yourself time and meditate to relieve yourself from everything that crowds your mind.

You may have lower urges if you are distracted or under a lot of pressure. Stress also affects your sexual behaviors.

Final Thoughts

Sexuality, including intimacy and sex, are a vital part of human nature. It can also have an impact on our overall health and well-being. It fulfills the feeling of belongingness and connection. However, untamed sexual urges can interfere with daily lives and relationships.

HOW TO CONTROL YOUR URGE TO HAVE SEX?

A good sex life is a very basic human need.

It often stands unmet, because of competitive lifestyles, leaving no room for personal gratification. In such cases, controlling your urge can become difficult. The following article will show you how you can do so.

1. Acceptance

The first step to control your sexual urges is to accept that there is no shame in feeling this way. Most societal norms deem these urges as moral depravity and force us to bury these feelings, instead of accepting it as a part of life. We are born to believe that sex is sin and sexual urges are an abomination. These urges are nothing but physical needs which only seek fulfillment, in some way or the other. Instinctually, man cannot abort sexual thoughts. With this acceptance and a strong desire to curb it, you can keep your feelings in control.

2. Triggers

The next step to controlling your sexual feelings is to know what sets them off. Admittedly, man is surrounded by sexual innuendoes and signs so obvious, that they are almost a part of our daily lives. When one is sexually satiated, these signs tend to pass by unnoticed, but in the face of sexual starvation, these signs end up titillating more than pacifying. Identifying these triggers will help keep the mind alert enough to steer clear of them.

3. Will Power

When it is considered that with enough will power, one can move a mountain, controlling sexual urges on the same plane should ideally be anyone's cup of tea. While it is impossible to obliterate sexual thoughts completely, curbing the intensity to a bare minimum will help you get through the day without distractions. A mental reminder, can serve as ample inspiration to help you power through the day without being tempted.

4. Transmutation

Translating your sexual urges to creative outputs will not only take your mind off them, but will help you make something new. At the end of the day, an urge is nothing but a feeling that enforces a lack of the desired object. Thus it is easy to manipulate with an equally engaging creative thought. Read a book, write poetry, paint or make pots. The end product of your misplaced creativity will provide equal satisfaction.

5. Exercise

Focusing your energy on something that consumes most of it and also helps you feel good, is a certain winner. Wake up early and go for a jog, or make swimming thrice a week a habit. You can also hit the gym every morning before work. .Whatever be the means, allow your body to get the much-required exercise to keep your mind more in control.

6. Seek Help

If nothing seems to get your mind off sex, this might be the start of a potential problem. If you are in a relationship, try to talk to your partner about these unmet needs. Maybe with regular intercourse, these urges will successfully be siphoned off. If not, then consult your doctor for psychological counselling to find a way out of these extensive urges. Obsessive thinking can be relieved with medication and therapy."This website uses cookies to ensure you get the best experience on our website. click here to review revised Privacy Policy."

HOW TO CONTROL SEXUAL DESIRE

When sexual desires and impulses arise within us at a very fast pace, we look for quick solutions to get rid of them. However, those solutions do not last for long, because it is not possible to control sexual desires through a quick fix. It requires thorough understanding, a lot of patience, internal steadiness, and most importantly, a firm commitment.

'Prevention is better than cure'
Prevention

By distancing yourself from the very things that cause the impulses in the first place. In other words, you should not look at images, watch videos, or read stories that are of a sexual nature. When you engage in any of these activities, they cause the multiplication of sexual impulses by tenfold, making it harder to control the desires.

Avoid any eye contact with people of the opposite sex and avoid touching at all costs. Avoid the company of people or friends that encourage sexuality, even jokingly. You never know when you might agree with them.

Let us see what advice and understanding Param Pujya Dadashri provides in His own words:

"As far as sex is concerned, the more one enjoys it, the more intense a burning desire will arise. Then sex will alight even more. Whatever happiness one enjoys, the thirst for it will increase. The thirst increases due to enjoyment. The thirst will go away by not indulging in it. That is called trushna (a thirst; strong desire). By not getting involved in the sexual act, one may become uneasy and unsettled for a month or two. However loss of familiarity is the key. With loss of familiarity, one will completely forget sexuality." He also advises you to, "Stay as far away from the company of those who are likely to trap you in sexuality, because if you get trapped even once, you will keep on getting into trap after trap. Therefore run! You must run as far away from that person as possible. You would not slip if you leave the place where there are chances of slipping."

In addition, prolonging sexual thoughts and fantasizing how you can enjoy it, will also make the impulses stronger. Therefore, a person should remain alert and not let any sexual thought continue for more than a second.

But how do you stop these thoughts or impulses in the first place? Through analysis and study of what sexuality actually is. This includes completely devaluing the object of attraction (i.e. the person, thoughts, body parts, etc.) to zero. You can do this by thinking about all the ways that the pleasure derived from sexuality is merely illusory, not real, and only temporary. When you are indulging in some form of sexuality, you tend to forget how filthy the human body actually is. For instance, you forget that every pore and opening in our body releases waste, which looks and smells awful. If faeces, sweat, and other discharge smell so bad, imagine how it would be inside the body. In addition, if there is real pleasure and happiness in physical contact and touch, then there should be pleasure even when your skin has an open wound or rash, but that is not the case. Furthermore, any form of dependency is the cause of suffering in this world, so how can dependency on someone else be the reason for happiness?

First Line of Defense

Once you have distanced yourself from sexuality and analyzed that there is no happiness in it, what do you when sexual impulses arise within you?

This is a list of tips and tricks on how to control sexual desires or impulses as soon as they arise:

Celibacy

Interrupt the link of sexual thoughts as soon as they arise in the mind. You can do this by changing the activity you are doing, changing your focus, thinking about some other work.

The moment any sexual thoughts arise within, pluck it immediately and throw it away. The plant of sex is the only one which if it becomes a little bigger, then it will not leave. Hence it needs to be pulled out from its very roots the moment it sprouts.

Picture the human body without skin. It is not a pretty sight. This practice is done not to create hatred, but to understand and get the real picture of the human body, so that we do not get attracted to it. If you make eye contact with anyone who arouses impulses of sexuality within you, you should immediately look away and change the inner visual link. Otherwise, the sexual seedling will grow. Therefore, it is best to eradicate it by asking for forgiveness immediately.

Ask for forgiveness by doing pratikraman for the desires that are occurring now and the ones that have occurred previously. The thoughts that are arising right now are sprouting from the knot of sexuality that was formed previously. Since this knot has not been removed, the thoughts will continue to come in some form.

If you get attracted to or are sexually tempted by a certain person, you have to ask for strength for practicing celibacy (brahmacharya) from the Soul of that person, by saying, 'O pure Soul! Give me the strength to maintain my celibacy (brahmacharya) with the entire world'. It is good if you ask for strength from Dada Bhagwan (the God within you), but it is best to ask directly from the Soul of the person towards whom you are attracted.

Apply Param Pujya Dadashri's unique key of Three Vision to stop any sexual impulses as soon as they arise. In this, three-step vision, one visualizes the person towards whom one is attracted, as naked in the first 'vision', without skin in the second 'vision', and with all the inner organs exposed in the third 'vision'. The aim of doing so is to see the non-Self complex, as it is. Once applied the person no longer remains a reason for attraction.

As soon as sexual impulses arise keep on reciting the following prayer: "Dear God! Give me infinite inner strength not to have, cause someone to have, nor encourage anyone to have any sexual desires, feelings, or gestures towards any living being, be it male, female, or of neutral gender. Give me the supreme strength to be free from all sexual desires, forever." The desires occur now because of our previous opinion that there is happiness in sexuality. By reciting the prayer above and asking for strength, we destroy the opinion and ask for the desires to not arise in the future.

Depending on the intensity and the type of impulses you have, you may need to use multiple keys at the same time or you may find some keys work better in some situations while others in other situations. Trick is not to get overwhelmed if one key does not work, you should be ready to use another key instantly. The battle is never lost; you just have to keep finding new ways of fighting.

Because of indifference towards sensual pleasures, the control (saiyam) over sexual desires and impulses that arise, will last forever. This indifference can only occur through detailed contemplation about how the happiness derived through sensual pleasures is only illusory. Rather than thinking about things that pull us more towards sexuality, we should think about all the consequences of being entrapped in sensual pleasures, and all the benefits and importance of brahmacharya (celibacy).

Feeling the urge to have sex is a normal part of human nature. However, these feelings can sometimes interfere with daily life and relationships, sometimes in a very detrimental way. Finding ways to control your sexual urges may help you improve your quality of life, your relationships, and your productivity. You can learn to avoid situations that make you have sexual urges. You can talk to others about your concerns, even seeking professional help if you feel your sexual urges are negatively impacting your life.

SEEKING IMMEDIATE SOLUTION

Get out of your current environment. Try to step away from any environment where you feel it's difficult to control your urges. If you are at home and feeling a compulsion to masturbate, for example, try taking a quick walk to the store. If you can't leave your current environment (if you're at work, for example), try talking to another coworker or taking a break.

It might also be helpful to have someone to help keep you accountable, such as a trusted friend or even a therapist.

Keep a to-do list in your pocket. Write down all the tasks, errands, or things around the house you need to do today. If you are feeling the need to engage in a compulsive behavior, look at your list and distract yourself with another activity.

If you think it is unlikely that you will be able to do something productive when you experience a strong sexual urge, then try to keep an easy distraction on hand, such as a good book or a puzzle you can work on.

Postpone your behavior until a later time. Putting off the compulsive behavior makes you think about your behavior before committing to it. It also helps you tolerate uncomfortable feelings and distress.

Set a time goal for yourself. Try telling yourself, "I'll watch porn in an hour," or whatever the largest amount of time you can commit to postponing may be. You may only be comfortable postponing your behavior for one minute. That's okay, give yourself one minute.

After your allotted time is up, you can choose to postpone again, or engage in your behavior. But choose to postpone whenever possible, even if it is just another minute.

After a while, you may be able to extend the amount of time you go without feeling the need to engage in the behavior.

Make a list of all of the negative consequences of your behavior. Making a list of all the risks or negative consequences associated with the behavior may help to stave off sexual urges as well. Write down all of the risks and potential consequences of acting on your behavior. Carry the list with you at all times and review it when you experience a sexual urge.

AVOID TRIGGERING SITUATIONS

Identify the triggers for your sexual urges. Spend some time thinking about your behavior and what leads you to have sexual impulses. Think about triggering stimuli, the time of day, as well as the environment in which you tend to have these urgings. See if there are any patterns that emerge in your behavior.

If you have discovered a pattern, figure out how you can break the cycle with new behaviors or lifestyle changes. For example, you may notice that you feel most overwhelmed with sexual urges in the evenings and on weekends -- when you are not working and don't have anything to do. You may decide to take up a new hobby in order to keep your mind off sex.

Perhaps you are triggered by stimuli in your environment. If you find yourself aroused by steamy love scenes in movies, for example, it may be best to watch other kinds of non-romantic films until you can get a better grip on your urges.

Consider keeping a journal of your actions and behavior leading up to sexual urges. A journal can help you identify triggers and patterns.

Avoid pornography. Pornography has turned into a billion-dollar industry, and viewing it is more acceptable than ever. This makes pornography difficult to ignore, but as it rewards sexual urges, it is best to avoid viewing it if you are prone to troublesome sexual urges. You may wish to put browser extensions or parental controls on your computer to make it difficult to access pornography on your computer. You could even have a friend or your partner install it and not inform you of the pass word.

Throw away any pornographic magazines, books, or movies you may have.

Consider avoiding masturbation. You may wish to avoid masturbating for a set amount of time to help you get your sexual urges under control. For some people, abstaining from masturbation may be more important than for others. You may wish to get suggestions about what would be appropriate for you from a therapist.

For example, if you feel you masturbate compulsively, it may be a good idea to commit to abstaining from masturbation for a set amount of time. This may also be appropriate if you have a porn addiction. For other people, masturbation may help you improve intimacy and improve your sexual health.

Abstain from drugs or alcohol. Drugs and alcohol can cause you to lose your inhibitions, including your sexual control. Stay away from parties and scenarios you think might be problematic.

Being under the influence of drugs and/or alcohol makes it more likely that you will engage in risky sexual activity.

Find effective methods to control your thoughts. Look for mental techniques you can use to help "change the subject" in your brain, when you begin to feel overwhelmed by sexual urges. You may wish to talk to a therapist about ways to manage obsessive thoughts. Some techniques may include:

Clearing your mind through meditation or mindfulness. Don't give up if this is very challenging at first! It is for most people. Have faith that it will get easier with practice. If you have a spiritual practice, you could also try prayer to help you focus your mind and get spiritual support.

Shifting your attention back to your present task. Acknowledge your sexual urges by telling yourself something like, "These are only thoughts. Right now they are not helping me, but hurting me." Then take a few deep breaths and shift your focus back to your current activity.

Minimize stress. Sometimes obsessive thoughts tend to creep up on you when you are feeling overwhelminly stressed. If you find this to be true for you with your sexual urges, figure out ways you can live a less stressful life.

For example, you may find yourself obsessively thinking about sex on days when you are running late for work. Experiment with earlier wake-up times or allowing extra commute time to see if your thought patterns change.

Make a list of various responsibilities you have and see what you can eliminate or delegate. Try to work smarter, not harder.

Keep yourself busy. Staying busy helps keep your mind preoccupied and focused on things other than sex. Take up a new hobby or fill your social calendar with activities with friends.

Channel your sexual energy into a creative project. Working through difficult emotions through one's imagination is a form of sublimation, or taking a "negative" or unwanted emotion and turning it into something more positive or useful.

Find a hobby that takes you away from triggering stimuli. For example, if you have a tendency to view porn at home alone, find a hobby that takes you out of the house and surrounds you with people, so that you are not in a triggering environment.

Exercise. Physical activity is one of the healthiest ways to control and manage a range of feelings and emotions, including the urge to have sex. Exercise regularly to combat sexual energy, or head to the nearest park or gym as soon as you start experiencing these feelings. Consider setting a fitness goal on which to focus. For example, you may decide to lose weight, lift a certain amount at the gym, or train for a race or long-distance bike ride. When you are not working out, you can spend time researching how to achieve your particular fitness goal, rather than be distracted by sexual urges.

Talking to Others Who Can Help You

See your doctor. Consider having an exam to rule out any physical problems that may be causing your sexual urges. Sometimes, illness or disorders can disrupt hormones and can make you feel hypersexual. Your doctor may ask you to see a psychologist or psychiatrist to get you evaluated for any mood disorders. For example, a high desire for sex is a symptom of bipolar disorder.

Be honest with your doctor about your sexual urges and express your concerns. Estimate how many times a day you think about sex or act on a sexual urge. For example, you might say, "I watch porn and masturbate four times a day." Your doctor can help you determine if your behavior is problematic or within the range of normalcy.

Talk to your partner about your feelings. If you are currently in a relationship, talk to your partner about your sexual urges. If you are feeling sexually unsatisfied in your relationship, be honest and discuss how the two of you could make an effort to prioritize sex.

You could say, "I am wondering if I am having so many urges because we haven't really been having sex lately. What do you think? Are you happy with our sex life?"

Understand that you and your partner may have different levels of sex drive. You may want to have sex more frequently than your partner. This doesn't make either of you wrong or right, it is just how you were made. Be honest with yourself and each other about if this can be managed or if this is a deal-breaker for the relationship.

Talk to your partner if you feel compelled to cheat on them. Be honest, even though it may be a difficult conversation. You could say, "I know this is painful to hear, but I am having sexual urges toward other people. I am telling you this because I want to be honest, and I am struggling."

Consider seeing a couples counselor with training in sexual addiction or sexual problems to help you navigate your relationship.

Talking to a trusted friend may also be a good option. They can help to hold you accountable for your goals, listen to you when you need to vent, and provide objective feedback.

Get a spiritual perspective. If you are concerned about controlling your sexual urges because of the faith you practice, consider seeking guidance from a spiritual leader in your faith community. Consider talking to clergy, a pastoral care leader, or a youth leader in your congregation.

Try not to be embarrassed. Most likely, leaders in your faith community have heard it all before and know how to address concerns. You could indicate your embarrassment when you ask to speak to them; for example, "I've been struggling with something kind of personal and embarrassing. Would there be a time I could talk to you in private about it?"

Ask your religious leader for resources that may be able to help you understand your struggle from a spiritual point of view.

SEEKING HELP FOR COMPULSIVE SEXUAL BEHAVIOR

Be aware of warning signs of sex addiction. Sex addiction, or compulsive sexual behavior, is considered such when your sexual urges and impulses begin to negatively impact your life. If you begin to feel overwhelmed by your sexual impulses, consider finding a counselor who can help you develop a treatment plan. Some warning signs to look out for include:

Considerable money spent finding ways to fulfill your sexual needs (for example, buying pornography, visiting strip clubs, or hiring sex workers)

Feeling driven to engage in sexual behaviors, but deriving no pleasure from them

Damage to interpersonal relationships, including those with intimate partners

Finding yourself having to apologize often for your behavior.

Engaging in risky sexual behaviors that can cause both physical and interpersonal problems (for example, having sex without a condom, or having sex with an employee).

Seek counseling. Consider finding a counselor who specializes in sexual addiction. To find a therapist, you may wish to consult your doctor, contact your employer's Employee Assistance Program, ask for a referral from your local community health agency, or do your own online research.

You may want to find a counselor who has a S-PSB (Specialist in Problematic Sexual Behaviors) or CSAT (Certified Sex Addiction Therapist) certification. These certifications show that the counselor has received training in sexual behavior causes and treatments

Therapists are trained to be open-minded, nonjudgmental, and accepting of other people's problems. Do not feel embarrassed or ashamed that you need to seek professional help. Therapists are also bound to confidentiality laws, and will protect your privacy, so long as you are not at risk of harming yourself or others, or you report abuse or neglect.10 Practical Ways to Battle Your Sexual Temptations. When someone confesses or is caught in an affair one of the first things they say is something to this affect, "I didn't mean it." Or "She/he meant nothing to me." In other words they end up in a place they never wanted to be. Most people don't set out to cheat on their spouse. It all starts small. It begins with a thought that goes uncontested, perhaps even nurtured into a fantasy. Those thoughts grow into an attitude and then the attitude grows into a disposition. That disposition erodes boundaries and clouds our sense of right and wrong.

This is difficult for most men. Our DNA is pre-loaded with the strong instinct to feel attraction and desire, yet life and morality demand that we are able to control those instincts. So how do we do that? For the sake of our marriages, relationships, or just spiritual well-being, we need to be able to find the answer. You are in a battle against sexual temptations and it's important to win early. Here are 10 ways to battle sexual temptation.

TEN PRACTICAL WAYS TO BATTLE YOUR SEXUAL TEMPTATIONS.

1. Avoid tempting situations.

Winning early means staying away from traps. The last thing you want to do is find yourself alone with the object of your unhealthy desires, whether it is images or actual people. If contact with that person is a must, then make sure it is always in a public space and others are around. Set boundaries surrounding your phone, the computer, and TV. Find a partner who is willing to help you with accountability.

2. Consider the consequences.
While pondering the object of your desire, also ponder the consequences of action. Is it going to help or hurt your marriage? How would your wife respond if she knew? Think about where your actions can lead and then imagine your wife finding out. Do you want to deal with the fallout? Always think of the end game. Where do you want to be? Are your thoughts and actions leading you there?

3. Avoid pornography.
Besides the obvious reasons that avoiding porn will help guard against lust, there are psychological reasons as well. Porn creates unrealistic expectations and desensitizes our minds towards our spouses. They can't possibly live up to what is viewed, and would we even want them to? This pushes the focus of your sexual desires outside of the home and can only lead to paths of destruction.

4. Use social media with caution.
There are many benefits of social media, but there are just as many pitfalls. We are reunited with people from our past and introduced to those who are new. Old sparks can be renewed or new ones can be lit.

For a married man, this can be extremely perilous. Always remain alert to true intentions when using social media.

5. Question your intent.

Most times, when our minds wander sexually, we aren't really seeking pure sex. We are seeking to replace something missing in our lives and our relationships. It could also be that we are trying to distract ourselves from dealing with something difficult. For each man, these things will be specific to his experiences. Figure out the root issue and work to correct it.

6. Practice sexual intimacy.

"When our minds and hearts are occupied in the right place, sexual lust has little room to operate. "While there is no way to go back to how you felt when your relationship was new, there are certainly plenty of ways to regain that level of relational excitement. Improving communication, date nights, passionate kissing and thoughtful gestures are just a few examples. When our minds and hearts are occupied in the right place, sexual lust has little room to operate.

7. Pray consistently.

Prayer is the act of communicating your thoughts, worries, hopes and dreams to God. Lift up the desires you are feeling and ask for help. God made you and knows you and can deliver you time and time again.

8. Choose your friends wisely.

When battling sexual temptation, there are plenty of people we can find that will encourage and enable it. You can still be their friend, but by all means, avoid joining them in their poor relational choices.

9. Keep high standards.
To be a gentleman is a choice. A very good choice, and this world today needs many more. Despite the vast amount of temptations that life throws our way, we should hold ourselves to the highest of moral standards. Self-discipline in all areas of our life leads to positive results.

10. Redirect your passion.
Rather than being controlled by untamed lust, direct that passion in positive directions. Use that energy to brainstorm about ways you can bless your wife. Perhaps focus on things that will make the world better like volunteering at a homeless shelter. Coach a youth sports team. Mentor troubled individuals.

Definition

Causes

Female reproductive system

Male reproductive system

Can a sex drive be too high?

How to lower libido.

Changes in sex drive, or libido, are normal. However, having a high sex drive can become a problem if it starts getting in the way of daily functioning.

It is important to note that there is no definition of a "normal" sex drive, and what one person sees as a high sex drive may seem normal to someone else.

Many people are curious about the nature of their sex drive. This article will explore some underlying causes of a high sex drive and provide some tips for controlling or reducing it.

What is sex drive?

A person's age and hormone levels may affect their sex drive.
Sex drive, otherwise known as libido, refers to a person's desire for sexual activity and arises from the basic biological need to reproduce.

It is a normal feeling that anyone can experience, whether a person wants to reproduce or not.

Levels of libido exist on a spectrum, from no desire for sex at all to wanting to engage in sexual activity very often.

Having a high sex drive is not a problem unless it excessively preoccupies a person's thoughts. For example, a person might wish to reduce their sex drive if it:

interferes with their work, social life, sleep, or health
affects their mental health
is difficult to feel satisfied, no matter how much sexual activity they have

affects the quality of their relationships

causes them to seek "risky" sex

Causes

What constitutes a normal sex drive differs for everyone, and people
are likely to desire sex more at different times in their lives.

Sex drive depends on factors such as:

Age
mental health status
energy levels
physical health status
relationship status
social interactions
medication, alcohol, or drug use
Age and hormones
Hormonal changes play a big role in sexual desire.

For young people, hormonal surges caused by puberty can trigger
feelings of sexual desire for the first time. Hormones will continue to
affect a person's libido throughout their life.

Some older research also suggests a possible association between
higher testosterone levels in men and having a higher sex drive.

Mental health

Stress levels can also influence how sexually charged a person feels.

In times of high stress, some people might feel low sexual desire,
while others might seek sexual satisfaction as a stress reliever.

Physical fitness and energy levels

ResearchTrusted Source has found that physically fit people are more likely to desire sex and enjoy heightened arousal and better orgasms.

Relationships

Having enjoyable sexual experiences, either with others or through masturbation, might also lead to an increased desire for sex. Intimacy between sexual partners has been shown to have a significant effectTrusted Source on the male sex drive.

On the other hand, if a person is unable to feel satisfied — either through a lack of sex or unsatisfying sexual experiences — their sex drive might also increase.

Substance use

Alcohol consumption lowers inhibitions, which might increase libido in the short term. However, alcohol dependency might decrease sexual arousal, performance, and satisfaction.

The use of stimulant drugs, such as cocaineTrusted Source, may also increase sexual desire but has links to increased "risky" sex in men who have sex with menTrusted Source and in young adultsTrusted Source.

The female reproductive system

Sexual desire can fluctuate throughout the menstrual cycle and often peaks around the time of ovulation. This is when testosterone levels are at their highest.

Ovulation is the time in the menstrual cycle when sperm can fertilize an egg. So, biologically speaking, it makes sense for females to feel more desire for sex around this time, as they are usually more likely to become pregnant.

For those acting on their increased sexual desire at this time but not wishing to become pregnant, it is especially important to use contraception carefully.

The male reproductive system
High testosterone levels are also linked to high sex drive in men. Testosterone production is usually at its peak at around 17 years of age, and levels tend to remain high for 2–3 decades after that.

This is also peak time for masturbation as an outlet for satisfying sexual desire. As men age, however, their testosterone levels tend to decrease, which can lead to a decrease in sexual desire.

Is it possible to have too high a sex drive?
Having a high sex drive only tends to become problematic when it gets in the way of other important aspects of life or if a person feels compelled to seek sexual activity in a way that feels out of control. This is known as compulsive sexual behavior.

Sometimes, when the libidos of sexual partners are not compatible, it can cause friction in the relationship.

How to lower libido

For anyone worried that their sex drive is very high and needs addressing, there are some strategies that might help.

The following are some things to try to lower sex drive:

Try talking therapy

If having a high sex drive is making a person unhappy, a counselor can help them explore their thoughts, feelings, and desires around sex.

They can help the person find ways to manage their sexual desire and any issues associated with it.

Try distraction

Engaging in sexual activities, either with a partner or through masturbation, is likely to perpetuate the need for more sex. So, if a person is keen to lower their sex drive, it may be worth trying not to act on every sexual impulse.

Distracting the mind with some form of physical exercise or an absorbing task might help a person channel this energy elsewhere.

Allow time for a relationship

People with a lower sex drive may misinterpret any intimate gesture by the other as a bid to have sex.

It may help to agree to be intimate without having sex. For example, go on a date or give each other a massage to show care for the other person — not so that they are more likely to agree to have sex.

Consider medication

If other strategies do not seem to work, it may be worth talking to a doctor about possible next steps.

Certain medications, such as antidepressants, may lower libido. A doctor may also suggest changing or lowering any current medications, if this is what is causing the increased arousal.

Doctors may also suggest consuming anaphrodisiacs — such as soy, licorice, hops, and various herbs — that may help lower libido.

6 reasons why you might have a high sex drive, or increased libido.

While a high libido is often considered healthy, sometimes you might wonder why your sex drive seems higher than normal or has suddenly increased.

Here are six reasons why your sex drive may feel unusually high:

1. Your hormone levels are changing

The sex hormones estrogen, progesterone, and testosterone levels can vary during your lifetime — but also within the course of a day — affecting your sex drive along with them.

For women, estrogen levels rise before and during ovulation, causing an increase in sex drive. Meanwhile, high testosterone levels in men have been linked to higher libido. High levels of testosterone are common in younger men and athletes using steroids.

A 2016 report found that being on estrogen therapies, like for menopause or bone loss, may be the reason for a higher sex drive in women. Additionally, if you're taking testosterone with low-dose estrogen therapy for postmenopausal purposes it may also heighten your sex drive.

2. You're going through puberty or aging

Those who are younger may have a higher sex drive than older adults. For example, testosterone production increases 10 times in adolescent boys, which explains the increase in arousal or interest in sex at that period in development.

However, middle-aged women may have a higher sex drive than younger women. A 2010 study of adult women found that people between 27 and 45 were more likely to think about sexual activities, have frequent sexual fantasies, a more active sex life, and more intense sexual fantasies than those aged 18 to 26.

3. You're exercising more

One reason your sex drive may be higher than usual is an increase in physical activity or weight loss. A small 2018 study revealed a positive relationship between physical fitness and a higher sex drive. In fact, the researchers found that in women, arousal was heavily influenced by cardiovascular endurance.

"Physical activity may make us feel more connected to our bodies and could increase self-image," says Kamil_Lewis, a sex and relationship therapist in Southern California. "When we feel good about ourselves, we're likely to want to engage in partnered sex more frequently."

4. You're in a healthy sexual relationship

Some people may experience a boost in libido if they find themselves in a sexual relationship that's more enjoyable than their past ones.

"If [sex is] a good and pleasurable experience, then it's going to make you want to do more of it. If it's a bad experience or it's not pleasurable, then a lot of times people will develop an aversion to sex," says Tamika K. Cross, MD, FACOG, an OBG-YN at Serenity_Women's Health & Med Spa in Pearland, Texas. "You're going to want more of something that feels good, and that's pleasurable to you."

5. You're less stressed

Your sex drive might be higher than usual because you're experiencing less stress. Higher stress levels release more cortisol — your fight or flight hormone — which can negatively impact your sex drive, says Cross.

In a small 2008 study, 30 women had their sex drives and cortisol levels measured before and after watching an erotic film. It found that women who had a decrease in cortisol had higher sex drives.

If you've recently noticed a dip in your stress levels, that may also explain an increase in sex drive. "Although sex is very physical, it's very mental and psychological as well," says Cross.

6. You've changed your medication

If you noticed a sudden change in libido it may be because you recently stopped using medication or decreased your dose. Antidepressants, in particular, can negatively impact your sex drive, says Cross. In a 2016 report, 40% of people experiencing sexual dysfunction could attribute it to antidepressant use.

Other medications that may hinder your sex drive include:

Anti-hypertensive medications, which are used to treat high blood pressure.

Therefore, if you recently stopped one of these medications, it might explain your higher than normal sex drive. Some people may prefer to discontinue or change a medication because it is impacting their sex life so significantly

Summary

For most people, having a high sex drive is a perfectly natural part of life that comes and goes depending on many factors.

It is usually nothing to worry about, but if it is causing stress or affecting other parts of life, it may be worth trying to channel this increased sexual energy into a different activity.

In extreme cases, a person can try seeking professional help.